ALZHEIMER'S DISEASE:

Your Questions Answered

ALZHEIMER'S DISEASE:

Yours Questions Answered

LIZ HODGKINSON

WARD LOCK

A WARD LOCK BOOK

First published in the UK 1995
by Ward Lock
Wellington House
125 Strand
LONDON
WC2R OBB

A Cassell Imprint

Distributed in the United States
by Sterling Publishing Co., Inc.
387 Park Avenue South, New York, NY 10016-8810

Distributed in Australia
by Capricorn Link (Australia) Pty Ltd
2/13 Carrington Road, Castle Hill NSW 2154

A British Library Cataloguing in Publication Data block for this book
may be obtained from the British Library

ISBN 0 7063 7401 0
Design and computer make-up by Tony & Penny Mills
Printed and bound in Great Britain by Biddles

Liz Hodgkinson is a journalist and author who has contributed to most leading
publications in the UK, including The Times, Guardian, Independent, Daily Mail, Cosmopolitan, and
Woman's Own. She broadcasts extensively on radio and television, has presented 'Woman's
Hour' and edits the magazine Top Woman. She is the author of more than 25 books on a
variety of subjects.

Contents

Introduction

Alzheimer's disease is an alarming and distressing condition in which sufferers first start to lose their memory, and then become progressively more forgetful and vacant; eventually they lapse into a state of complete apathy where they no longer have any real connection with the world around them. Nevertheless they may go on living for many years in an increasingly twilight and meaningless condition.

Although Alzheimer's is the most usual name, the condition is also known as pre-senile dementia and Dementia of the Alzheimer's Type (DAT). In the USA, Alzheimer's is usually known as DAT, while, in the UK, the term Alzheimer's remains more common.

Alzheimer's is a disease which everyone dreads, as it is characterized by confusion, senility and, eventually, total deterioration of personality. It is also the commonest cause of pre-senile and senile dementia.

Not long ago, Alzheimer's was considered a shameful complaint and families tried to keep their suffering relatives hidden. It was regarded as a kind of mental illness, akin to schizophrenia or mental retardation.

Now, thanks to pioneering research, carried out mainly in the USA and the UK over the past few years, we know that Alzheimer's is not a mental condition at all but a physical disease in which the brain cells progressively and irreversibly deteriorate.

For some reason not yet fully understood a certain protein accumulates in the tissues and cells of the brain, causing them to become disorganized and die. In normal conditions this protein, known as β-amyloid protein, can be effectively processed and rendered ineffective by the immune system.

When Alzheimer's sets in, this protein can no longer be processed, and, although it is not living matter, it has much in common with a virus. Because Alzheimer's affects the brain, and eventually the emotions, character and behaviour, it has much in common with mental illness and mental retardation, and is often mistakenly considered to be a mental rather than a physical condition.

Indeed, it eventually becomes indistinguishable in

its effects from a mental illness. At the moment, despite the many theories, nobody knows exactly what causes the brain cells to become disorganized in this fashion when some people reach a certain age. Some researchers have proposed that aluminium, a metal which affects the nervous system, may be to blame but the fact is that no theories have so far hardened into fact, and the aluminium theory, along with many others concerning Alzheimer's, remains controversial.

All we know about Alzheimer's is that, at present, there is no way to prevent or cure the complaint. Nor is any effective medical treatment available. Once the condition sets in, the decline may be slow or it may be rapid, but it is definitely irreversible. There is no way to 'get the person back' after a diagnosis of Alzheimer's. It is this which caused people to question the veracity of former Guinness chairman Ernest Saunders who was released from prison on the grounds that he was suffering from Alzheimer's disease

On his release, he appeared to make a full recovery, which is clearly impossible. It seems more likely that Saunders was suffering from deep depression, which can have symptoms in common with Alzheimer's, the difference being that depression can be treated and people can recover, whereas there is no recorded case of anyone recovering from Alzheimer's. But, to give Saunders the benefit of the doubt, a diagnosis of Alzheimer's is very often an inspired guess rather than a completely accurate assessment of the situation. It is possible that his doctors made a mistake.

However, the fact that the disease is irreversible does not mean that nothing can be done. Although there is still no effective treatment, our improved knowledge of the disease means that its sufferers are more likely to be cared for with humanity and compassion. It is always tragic to see a much-loved and once-lively person descend into the twilight zone of Alzheimer's, but expert help is now available for carers and, with greater understanding, better care can be given to those who are afflicted with this condition.

There are many ways in which the burden on carers can be lifted, but the condition must first be admitted and understood. Many aspects of the sufferers' behaviour become less frightening and anxiety-making once it is realized that they cannot help being ill and their behaviour cannot be altered. The condition is physical, the result of deterioration of the brain cells, and is most certainly not due to the person deliberately becoming crochety or difficult.

Because of the amount of research now being conducted into Alzheimer's on both sides of the Atlantic and in Australia, we can expect that before long, an effective treatment may become available. Even if the dead brain cells cannot be brought back to life, scientists hope that they may soon discover a way of preventing existing cells from becoming damaged and dying. Once the mechanisms responsible for the damage are more fully understood, there is hope for the development of a drug which will be able to halt the worse excesses of the disease.

Alternatively, a way may be found to prevent the build-up of β-amyloid protein in the first place. One problem is that no one knows who may be at risk. Alzheimer's descends without warning and there is, at the moment, no way of knowing in advance who it will affect. That is why it comes as such a nasty shock – and why few people are prepared for it when it enters their lives.

No one expects to get Alzheimer's – but no one is guaranteed to be immune either. What we do know is that Alzheimer's is no respecter of persons. It has nothing to do with personality, character or lifestyle.

Many notable people have suffered from

Alzheimer's, e.g. Sir Winston Churchill, Rita Hayworth and the children's writer Enid Blyton. Recently, ex-President Reagan of the USA publicly stated that he may himself be suffering from Alzheimer's. This contrasts markedly with the situation about three decades ago when, for 15 years, the fact of Churchill's gradually worsening mental state through Alzheimer's was kept carefully hidden from the public.

In some ways, the growth of public awareness of Alzheimer's has mirrored that of cancer. About 20 years ago, there were no books on cancer other than those aimed at the medical profession, and the word 'cancer' was hardly ever mentioned in public. Doctors hid diagnoses from sufferers and their families and, because of all this secrecy, cancer was considered an unmentionable disease. Until recently, Alzheimer's was regarded in the same light, but attitudes are changing.

Alzheimer's is not contagious and, although there may sometimes be a genetic component to the disease, it does not seem to run in families. It is a disease primarily of old age, just like arthritis or osteoporosis.

The heaviest burden falls mostly on the carers, usually the immediate family or partner. Initially, the person with the disease may have only a very hazy idea of what is happening, and this will certainly be the case eventually. Because the brain is not fully functional, and becomes less so as time goes on, the sufferers themselves are often spared the worst realizations of what is happening to them. Onlookers, though, feel sad, helpless, and even angry at the disintegration of a previously much-loved individual.

The story of Rita Hayworth is one example of the progress of the disease. Rita, one of the most dazzling Hollywood stars of the 1940s and 1950s, died in 1987 from Alzheimer's. Although there had been some early warning signs, Alzheimer's was not definitely diagnosed until 1980, when she was 60 years old. Before then, people had erroneously gained the impression the she was drunk, or perhaps on drugs.

Although she was known to be an alcoholic, alcohol did not appear to be the cause of the disease and her daughter, Princess Yasmin, has said that her mother never drank after she checked into hospital. Nobody suspected Alzheimer's.

During the first stages of the illness, Rita was able to cope on her own, but soon became confused and forgetful of where she was. Her daughter has described the heartbreak of watching her once beautiful mother gradually sink into the permanent confused state which characterizes the disease. On some days, apparently, Rita would become very angry, and no one could discover why. Her speech became a meaningless mumble and she constantly shuffled her hands and feet. She could not bear to watch television and her daughter would play music for her instead. In some sad photographs during her decline, Rita was photographed looking dishevelled and acting aggressively.

Princess Yasmin, daughter of Rita and Prince Aly Khan, says that she wants to continue raising money for research in the hope that somebody will come up with a cure. This she does by holding Rita Hayworth balls and galas, and these occasions on behalf of the Alzheimer's Association in the USA have been instrumental in raising funds to carry out pioneering research.

This book gives all the up-to-date information about Alzheimer's, and explains how this very specific disease differs from normal ageing, and also from certain other conditions that may affect older people, e.g. depression or anxiety.

Questions and Answers

1 Alzheimer's Disease

Q Why is the condition called Alzheimer's disease?

The condition we now know as Alzheimer's disease was first identified in 1906 by a German neurologist, Alois Alzheimer. He gave his name to the disease after describing, in a medical paper, changes in the brain tissue of a patient who had died after suffering from confusion, apathy and memory loss.

Under the microscope, Dr Alzheimer noted a disorganization in the nerve cells, which he called 'neurofibrillary tangles' and accumulations of debris, which he termed 'senile plaques'. It seemed that it was these changes which were responsible for the memory loss so overwhelmingly characteristic of Alzheimer's.

At the time, neither he nor anyone else knew what might be causing the plaques and tangles and, since his day, research has been aimed along these lines. Although far more is understood about the disease these days, no satisfactory answer has yet been obtained.

What exactly are 'neurofibrillary tangles' and 'senile plaques'?

All human brain tissue contains millions of nerve cells with thread-like extensions called nerve-fibres. In Alzheimer's, the normally well-ordered arrangement of the nerve cells becomes wildly disorganized – hence the term 'neurofibrillary tangles' – and affected cells stop functioning; part of the brain dies and cannot be brought back to life. As time goes on, more brain cells die and, as they do so, patients deteriorate further.

The structures known as senile plaques are accumulations of debris surrounding a central core of b-amyloid peptide, a protein derivative found in the brain. β-amyloid is a small fragment of a complex protein, which, for some reason, accumulates in nerve tissue and destroys it.

Senile plaques and neurofibrillary tangles, for some reason not yet known, affect only those parts of the brain concerned with memory and retention of information. This kind of brain deterioration is very serious because the nerve cells that are being systematically destroyed are those that are most essential to the proper functioning of the muscles as well as the production of hormones, which affect the emotions. Nerve tissues affected by Alzheimer's look dead and lifeless.

Q How are these plaques and tangles seen?

They can only be seen under the microscope when brains of Alzheimer's sufferers are examined during a post-mortem examination. There is no way of examining them in living people but, in any case, there is little that can be done to reverse the process of deterioration once it has begun.

In many cases, Alzheimer's can only be accurately diagnosed after the patient is dead and it is from post-mortem examinations of brain cells that most of the advances and understanding of Alzheimer's have come about.

Q Do other species suffer from Alzheimer's?

No, it appears not. In some animals, for instance dogs and certain primates, changes in the brain occur with age, but these are not the same as in Alzheimer's.

Q **Are these plaques and tangles found in conditions other than Alzheimer's?**

Yes. To some extent they are part of normal ageing. They are also found in the brains of people suffering from Down's syndrome. The brains of some old people may show these changes although there have been people in their 80s and 90s in whom no traces of this kind of deterioration have been found.

There will be evidence of plaques and tangles in the brain cells of most people over 70 years old but, unless these people have Alzheimer's, they will not significantly affect thinking, memory or other aspects of brain function.

It was once thought that the condition we now recognize as Alzheimer's was something to be expected as people got older. We now know that it is an abnormal condition and cannot be considered part of the process of ageing. It is a disease process, like arthritis, but, unlike arthritis there is no remission.

Q **Is there a connection between Down's syndrome and Alzheimer's?**

Yes, to the extent that the same kind of tangles and

plaques are found in the brains of both Down's syndrome and Alzheimer's sufferers. Down's syndrome is associated with a certain form of mental retardation and a characteristic physical appearance, and the condition is the result of a chromosome abnormality. All Down's syndrome sufferers have an extra chromosome and it has been suggested that this may be the case in a very small proportion of Alzheimer's sufferers.

Post-mortem examinations of the brains of Down's syndrome sufferers show that, in most cases, the plaques and tangles are so numerous that they may be indistinguishable from those in an Alzheimer's sufferer. The main difference is that, in cases of Down's syndrome, these changes occur very much earlier, probably before the age of 40 years. At the moment, though, research into the link between Alzheimer's and Down's is at a very early stage and no firm conclusions can be drawn.

Another important difference is that Down's cases suffer from mental retardation from birth, whereas Alzheimer's sufferers have normal intelligence and functioning until the disease develops.

What we do know, however, is that like Alzheimer's disease, Down's syndrome is not preventable or curable. In the old days, people with Down's syndrome did not live for much longer than 30 years. Better medical and social care now enables some people with Down's to live to quite old ages and it is because of this that their brains can usefully be compared with those of Alzheimer's sufferers.

Q **Alzheimer's is often called pre-senile dementia. What is the difference between this and senile dementia?**

The difference is really a matter of the age of on-set of the dementia. Nowadays, for practical purposes, the condition is often referred to as Alzheimer's disease, or pre-senile dementia, when the onset of the illness occurs before the age of 65 years, and senile dementia when the age of onset is much later.

In post-mortems, the brain changes found in Alzheimer's disease and senile dementia are almost exactly the same. They are, in fact, the same disease. Whatever the age of onset, the disease process appears to follow the same course but Alzheimer's is particularly devastating because it affects people who could still be considered as in their prime.

With Alzheimer's, too, the symptoms are more severe and the progress of the disease much swifter. The earlier a person contracts Alzheimer's, the shorter the life expectancy.

Q What does it actually mean to have Alzheimer's?

Alzheimer's is the term used for progressive loss of mental function and can be defined as a generalized and gradual impairment of memory, intellect and personality with no loss of consciousness. There are insidious and sometimes irreversible changes in three areas: behaviour, mood, and thought processes.

Initially there are occasional lapses of memory, although everyone experiences these to some extent and they are not necessarily an indication of Alzheimer's. Memory loss turns into a disease when it becomes not only progressively worse but also irreversible.

Indeed, the loss of short-term memory is the most outstanding characteristic of Alzheimer's and, for some time after the disease has set in, long-term memory remains intact.

However, all long-term memory starts off as

short-term memory and, eventually, there seems to be no memory at all. Before long, no new information can be assimilated. There comes a time when Alzheimer's patients forget everything, even the most familiar names and faces. They no longer recognize their nearest and dearest, they cannot carry on a conversation, and they spend their days staring into space, no longer able to read a newspaper, listen to the radio or television or carry on a conversation. There may be some daily or day-to-day fluctuations but, on the whole, there are no periods of remission.

The saddest thing is that people can live for years in this state and they usually die of some other illness, e.g. pneumonia, rather than Alzheimer's.

Q How common is Alzheimer's?

It is estimated that about 700,000 people in the UK suffer from Alzheimer's, and between 3 and 4 million in the USA. So, although it is not all that rare, neither is it all that common.

Q Is it on the increase?

It does not seem to be. Although there *appear* to be more cases of Alzheimer's than there used to be, this is probably because of increased public awareness, and the far higher profile which the disease now has. Also, with the improvement in diagnostic techniques, more accurate diagnoses are now being made.

Another reason for the apparent increase is that people are now living longer than at any other time in history. As Alzheimer's rarely occurs before the age of 60 years, the more people living beyond this age, the more common it will become. Also, because of the better care available, Alzheimer's patients are likely to live longer than they have in the past.

Q Are men or women more affected?

Alzheimer's disease appears to affect both men and women equally. There appears to be no link with intelligence levels, education or achievement, race or geographical distribution of the illness. The sole common factor is that it affects mainly older people.

Q Is memory loss always an indication of Alzheimer's?

No, there can be a number of reasons for memory loss. Although people often appear to be more forgetful as they get older, it is not always realized that young people can also be forgetful. So forgetfulness should not just be associated with getting older – it is a condition which can persist throughout life.

Sometimes, memory loss may result from the effects of anaesthesia – older people may take a long time to recover from surgery or other operations – injury, or medication. It is when all these possibilities have been ruled out, and when memory loss is new and disturbing, that Alzheimer's may be suspected. This is why, when serious lapses of memory occur in older people, other factors must be ruled out before a diagnosis of Alzheimer's can be made.

The point about Alzheimer's and other dementing illnesses is that the memory loss is permanent, and not mere forgetfulness. For example, sufferers may go shopping several times for the same things, and will pay bills that they have already paid. It is as if the slate of their memory is constantly being wiped clean, this is very different from going downstairs to fetch something and forgetting what you are supposed to be fetching.

With Alzheimer's, the memory loss is such that the sufferer appears to be living in a different world from the rest of us.

Q What does 'dementia' mean? Do sufferers become demented in the usual sense of the word?

Not really. The term dementia is misleading, as it is simply used to describe the progressive loss of mental functions. It does not mean that sufferers become 'demented' in the sense that they flail around, scream and shout. In fact, they behave in just the opposite fashion, becoming apathetic, listless and largely unaware of what is going on around them.

Sometimes, there may be worrying personality changes, (e.g. hostility, suspicion and aggression) but these are usually short-lived and are characteristic of the disease. As time goes on, and the dementia becomes progressively worse, sufferers become increasingly apathetic and loss of personality sets in. Eventually, they become completely unrecognizable as the individuals they once were, however lively, bright and vivacious that was.

Q Can Alzheimer's be considered a psychological or psychosomatic disease?

No, it has nothing to do with personality, emotions or character. There is no particular personality type which is more likely to succumb to Alzheimer's than another and it has nothing to do with any mental condition, even though sufferers are liable to display distressing emotional reactions, such as excessive weepiness, bad temper and paranoid tendencies.

Alzheimer's is essentially a physiological disease and it has its roots in a physical malfunction. Because it affects the brain, and therefore mental functioning, it has psychological implications but it does not have a psychiatric origin, although it is sometimes treated as a psychiatric disease.

Some authorities consider that many 'mental' illnesses have physical causes, e.g. the failure of certain essential minerals and vitamins to reach the brain. This appears to be the case with hyperactive children and has been put forward as a cause of schizophrenia. Deficiencies of zinc and other essential minerals are also known to result in mental and emotional problems. But we do not yet know what causes the brain to go wrong in cases of Alzheimer's.

What is amyloid protein?

This is the name given to deposits of abnormally aggregated protein molecules. These proteins, known technically as β-amyloid protein peptides, were discovered in the early 1980s, and are derived from another type of protein, known as amyloid precursor protein (APP) which is found in every cell of the human body.

In normal circumstances, APP is thought to have some rôle in nerve cell growth and possibly in the transmission of messages from one cell to another. Currently, however, this is all speculative and the exact role of APP is unknown.

Experiments are now in progress to establish the exact rôle of APP in normal cell function, so that the abnormalities seen in Alzheimer's can be more fully understood.

How is amyloid precursor protein (APP) related to Alzheimer's?

Some of the understanding about APP comes from studies of people with Down's syndrome. It has been known for some time that Down's sufferers have three chromosomes 21 whereas most people have only two. It is this extra chromosome which causes the characteristic appearance and mental retardation of Down's syndrome sufferers.

Should they live long enough, Down's sufferers will almost certainly develop Alzheimer's in their 40s or 50s. This may be due to the extra gene which they have for APP causing an increased production of β-amyloid protein peptide, this is then deposited in the brain – and cannot get out.

It seems, from research carried out so far, that APP is linked to the onset of Alzheimer's, but many questions remain and far more research needs to be done.

All we know at present it that the plaques and tangles found in the brains of Alzheimer's sufferers are similar to those found in Down's syndrome cases. There may, or may not be a direct link between the conditions. Even though much is now known about the brain and how it functions normally, diseases of the brain are by no means fully understood.

Q What is the difference between Alzheimer's and the ordinary ageing process?

At first, there may seem no difference because old

people often appear to be forgetful and find difficulty in assimilating new information. In cases of Alzheimer's, however, the deterioration is irreversible and there are no remissions. Also, there are particular kinds of memory loss associated with Alzheimer's that do not appear in ordinary ageing, such as forgetting all familiar faces, even that of the partner.

With the ordinary ageing process, whatever else happens, memories of long ago are always retained. With Alzheimer's, eventually everything is lost beyond recall.

 ## What happens to Alzheimer's sufferers?

Behaviour is affected as sufferers becomes muddled and restless, with distracted behaviour that has no apparent reason. There may be few signs of interest or initiative and sufferers becomes dull and listless. They may also show antisocial behaviour, such as uninhibited sexual behaviour or shoplifting. They may also develop meaningless but obsessive rituals, for example constant hand washing, touching of door knobs or fiddling with certain objects. In the latter stages of the disease, there may be complete disorientation, incoherence and incontinence. Some sufferers may start wandering, especially at night.

Thought processes slow down and become reduced in content. There may be some element of persecution mania involving the partner or other carers. As time goes on, there may be difficulty in understanding abstract ideas and the same ideas may be repeated over and over again. Impaired judgement may put the person into a dangerous situation, e.g. when driving.

Here is the story of a typical Alzheimer's victim. Sid, at 60 years old, seemed to be in good health and enjoyed his work as a local government officer in the rating department of a large London borough. When the community tax replaced the rating system Sid appeared to be confused about how it was to take place. He seemed unable to understand the processes involved and this bothered his supervisors, as Sid had always been particularly alert before. However, they put it down to the fact that he was getting old and having difficulty in taking on new ideas.

A few weeks later, he forgot on a couple of occasions to pick up some shopping which his wife had asked him to collect. He then completely forgot that his son and daughter-in-law were coming to stay for the weekend. When they arrived, he went to the pub for drink with some friends and, when he came back, he had once again forgotten that his son and daughter-in-law were there.

Sid's wife later became alarmed when she found him writing out cheques to pay bills which had already been paid. She pointed out the cheque stubs to him, but it was clear that Sid had no recollection of ever paying those particular bills.

Worried, she asked him to see a doctor, as his memory appeared to be getting increasingly worse. Reluctantly, he agreed and the doctor carried out some brain function tests. The results were normal and the doctor prescribed anti-depressant pills, thinking perhaps that Sid had become affected by the changes at work.

The pills had no effect and Sid's memory got worse and worse. In addition he started to become paranoid, convinced he was being spied on and that people were watching him through the walls. He was still going to work but, by now, other people were doing most of his job. He became increasingly vacant and spent most of his time sitting in his chair, staring into space. Occasionally, he would have bursts of bad temper, which were quite alien to his previous calm character. After a couple of years, Sid's boss called his wife and said that, in his opinion, Sid was incapable of carrying on the job any longer. He was now 62 years old and could, therefore, retire, if he wanted to.

Sid's wife persuaded him to take early retirement, after which he spent most of the time sitting at home staring into space. He would boil a kettle for a cup of tea and then forget he had done it. Occasionally he would go for a walk, but he seemed unable to hold a conversation with his old friends. He promised his wife that he would not drive but, every now and again, he would take the car out, until she finally insisted on having the keys all the time.

His wife, by now getting desperate, took him to see another doctor, who carried out more tests. A computerized axial tomography (CAT) scan showed that his brain had shrunk considerably in size and this doctor diagnosed Alzheimer's, saying that there was no known cure or treatment for the condition.

Sid could no longer be left at home, and his wife and son tried to get him into a home, or arrange proper nursing care – he was now considered beyond ordinary care. The trouble was, all the nursing homes that would take him cost far more than they could afford.

Eventually, they found a home after Sid's son had agreed to contribute to the weekly fees. The home was well set up to care for Alzheimer's sufferers, and they did their best for his worsening condition. Before long, Sid no longer recognized his wife, son or daughter-in-law when they came to see him and he stopped talking altogether. He became progressively weaker and lived for 18 months after going into the nursing home. He died, not of Alzheimer's, but of pneumonia.

Although this story is fairly typical, it refers to a specific case and the disease will not follow an identical progression in every sufferer. Most aspects, however, will be broadly similar, particularly the devastation caused to families because of the feeling of utter helplessness.

 Who is most at risk?

Anybody can fall victim to Alzheimer's. It is no respecter of persons and has no link with intelligence, class, education or occupation. A Swedish study carried out in 1992 suggested that 50 per cent of all cases had a cardio-vascular cause and that the prevention of such problems could significantly reduce the incidence of dementia.

The researchers screened nearly 500 85-year olds,

giving them physical examinations and scans. One-third of these cases had dementias. Of these, 43 per cent had dementia of cardiovascular origin and the rest due to other causes. The authors of this report, which appeared in the *New England Journal of Medicine*, concluded that dietary changes, stopping smoking, aspirin therapy and treatment of high blood pressure could do a lot to prevent the disease.

This, however, is the only study of its type and there have been no follow-ups. There have been no further reliable studies to show a link between smoking and the onset of dementias, and there is little else to suggest that heart problems could aggravate or cause the condition.

As to dietary changes, (see also page 52), the evidence remains highly speculative. So far, there have been no other studies to suggest a link between lifestyle and the onset of dementias. We know that Sir Winston Churchill, who developed Alzheimer's in his final years, was a highly self-indulgent eater, smoker and drinker, but whether this contributed to the onset of the disease is unknown.

Certainly, there are many people who suffer from dementias in their later years who have never smoked or drank and do not have high blood pressure so, as yet, no conclusions can be drawn.

Q Does anything spark off Alzheimer's?

No, there are no known precipitating factors, although it often seems to follow a bad bout of influenza, or other viral illness. It also does not appear to follow emotional trauma, e.g. bereavement, divorce or other serious loss.

Q How easy is Alzheimer's to diagnose?

Diagnosis is not easy because forgetfulness, memory loss and dementia are symptoms of a number of diseases. There are also a number of brain diseases which are associated with progressive dementia and, in some cases, a diagnosis may be a matter of guesswork.

Brain diseases which may follow a similar pattern to Alzheimer's are described below.

1. Pick's Disease, which is much rarer than Alzheimer's, follows a similar pattern, but the appearance of tangles and plaques under the microscope is quite different. This has led researchers to believe that, when effective treatments are found, those for Alzheimer's and Pick's diseases will be different. Pick's sufferers overeat, they may become sexually hyperactive and mindlessly euphoric. They

will stuff anything, edible or not, into their mouths, and will even try to eat matches, rubber bands, toilet paper.

2. Normal-pressure hydrocephalus (NPH) used to be known as 'water on the brain' and involves impaired circulation of the spinal fluid and destruction of the brain tissue. Progress of the disease is usually rapid and sufferers will have a history of injury to the brain. NPH produces disturbances in walking and standing, and causes incontinence. It is one of the few treatable types of dementia – surgery may be effective – and needs to be excluded before one can proceed with an accurate diagnosis of Alzheimer's.

3. Huntington's disease (formerly known as Huntington's chorea) can be easily diagnosed from the peculiar writhing movements of the sufferer, so is unlikely to be confused with Alzheimer's.

4. Creutzfeldt-Jakob disease is caused by a slow virus and runs a fairly rapid course. It is similar to Alzheimer's in that there is a slightly abnormal accumulation of protein.

5. Wilson's disease causes progressive dementia,

but is a rare illness associated with liver disease.

6. Lewy body disease is becoming increasingly recognized and is probably the second most common cause of dementia after Alzheimer's disease.

Age is one of the most important factors in the accurate diagnosis of Alzheimer's disease. Any dementia which begins earlier than age 60 years is unlikely (except in cases of Down's syndrome) to be Alzheimer's. The most common way of diagnosing Alzheimer's is to give the sufferer a series of psychological and behavioural tests.

Q What do these of tests consist of?

Doctors may ask sufferers, or suspected sufferers, a series of simple questions, such as where and when they were born, what day of the week it is, where they are, the name the Queen, which country they are living in, and which party is in power. These are the kind of questions to which everyone should know the answer. If the interviewee becomes confused by them, then dementia may be suspected.

A similar test, designed to measure intelligence quotients (IQ) and known as the Wechsler Adult

Intelligence Scale, asks another series of simple questions, (for example, How many wings does a bird have? In what way are a lion and tiger alike?) and a number of simple memory questions.

There are a number of other psychological questionnaires which test intelligence and memory levels, and these are the commonest ways in which a diagnosis of dementia is made.

Q Are there scientific instruments or techniques which can aid diagnosis?

Yes. An electro-encephalograph (EEG) measures brain wave activity by recording voltage patterns generated in the brain and this can give some clues. In Alzheimer's sufferers, brain rhythms are considerably slowed down and the changes are most noticeable in the areas of the brain connected with memory.

Cerebrospinal fluid examination may also be carried out by doctors during the early stages of diagnosis. This is a routine procedure involving little more than the prick of a needle.

X-rays are of little use in diagnosing Alzheimer's as they provide an image of the skull rather than the brain. The computerized axial tomography

(CAT) scan is the most important diagnostic test that doctors can carry out. This scan outlines the brain and enables doctors to see small injuries, e.g. strokes or tumours. As with other tests, however, the unmistakeable signs of Alzheimer's only show up on a CAT scan when the disease is fairly advanced, so it is unable to confirm the illness in its early stages.

Scientists in the USA have discovered that eye drops used in eye examinations produce a hyper-sensitive reaction in those with Alzheimer's and, according to initial tests, this appears to be 95 per cent accurate as a diagnosis.

Doctors at the Radcliffe Infirmary in Oxford, UK, have found that X-ray computed tomography and single photon emission computed tomography – both sophisticated forms of brain scan – may provide an indication of Alzheimer's.

A genetic test which estimates the likelihood of Alzheimer's disease developing in those with Down's syndrome has been developed jointly in the USA and the UK. It is adapted from DNA fingerprinting and, according to researchers, could be used in foetuses to predict the likelihood of Alzheimer's in later life.

The main value of tests and scans is to eliminate other illnesses, rather than to provide a positive diagnosis of Alzheimer's. Some brain illnesses are treatable, so it is always worth having these tests.

The only absolute way of diagnosing Alzheimer's is still by examination of the brain at autopsy. Many doctors believe that a diagnosis of Alzheimer's is still only a clinical opinion, and that this situation is likely to remain for the foreseeable future.

In general, doctors still rely on psychological tests and behavioural observations rather than sophisticated equipment for the diagnosis of Alzheimer's. However, the search is on for a simple early test which will enable people to benefit from treatment options and to prepare themselves for the worsening time ahead.

Q Are there any early warning signs of Alzheimer's?

Not usually. The disease strikes without warning and its course may be slow or rapid. But a memory loss which is never restored and which gets progressively worse is the major sign.

Q How does Alzheimer's differ from depression?

At first, it may not be possible to distinguish between depression, which is not usually long term, and Alzheimer's, which is. Old people are sometimes diagnosed as suffering from Alzheimer's, and treated as such, when they are really seriously depressed. Confusingly, depression is a feature of most dementing illnesses, at least at some stages.

It is important to differentiate between the two because depression may well be treatable through the use of suitable drugs, psychotherapy or group therapy.

Depression is usually diagnosed when mood changes or reactions to events are more extreme or longer lasting than would normally be expected. It is common after the death of a spouse or other close relative but, in these cases, the mood will lift after a while, although severe depression may come back from time to time.

Common symptoms of depression are:

1. Mood swings.

2. Memory loss.

3. A bad mood in the morning which often lifts during the day.

4. Awareness of the problem.

5. Use of drugs, alcohol, food or nicotine for relief.

In contrast, the most common symptoms of dementia are:

1. An even decline over months or years, with no let-up or lightening of mood.

2. Attempts to hide memory loss.

3. The illness appearing to get worse, rather than better, as the day wears on and the sufferer becomes tired.

4. Complete unawareness of the disability.

5. No attempt being made to improve mood by resorting to drugs, alcohol, food or nicotine.

It must be said that doctors do not always appreciate the difference between dementia and depression, and may treat inappropriately. It can also be easy to mistake the apathy due to depression for dementia, especially nowadays, when Alzheimer's or some other dementia is often suspected although it is not actually present.

Q Do only old people suffer?

Alzheimer's mostly affects those over 60 years old but, in some rare instances, it can affect people in their 30s, 40s and 50s. Alzheimer's becomes increasingly common with increasing age.

Q Can Alzheimer's be inherited?

In some cases, it seems so. Scientists have discovered that people who succumb to Alzheimer's early in life – say in their 40s or 50s – often have a genetic predisposition to the disease. But Alzheimer's may have a genetic component anyway. Research is certainly proceeding along these lines.

Q Aluminium has been associated with Alzheimer's. What is the evidence for this?

The link between aluminium and Alzheimer's is still the subject of controversy. Professor John Edwardson at the neuro-chemical pathology unit of Newcastle-upon-Tyne General Hospital was the first to study this. His research team observed that, in the brain tissue of Alzheimer's sufferers from areas supplied with water that had been treated for high peat content, there were traces of aluminium. The next stage was to determine how this metal could cross the blood-brain barrier and Professor Edwardsons' work showed that aluminium could become bound to an important molecule in the blood, known as transferrin.

In support of this theory, it was noted that, in the early days of renal dialysis, kidney patients used to take in excess aluminium and appeared to be at far higher risk of developing Alzheimer's than people taking it in from the water supply. There is also some evidence that people who receive a lot of injections are at greater risk of developing Alzheimer's because of the aluminium content of the hypodermic syringe.

The aluminium theory developed because one of the most consistent findings in post-mortems was an excess of aluminium in the brain. In most victims, however, the amounts of extra aluminium were extremely small and could be detected only by the most sensitive instruments. Other researchers found that aluminium tends to collect in brains of older people anyway, whether or not they succumb to Alzheimer's. Aluminium has no known biological function in human beings and, in any case, the excess found in the brains of Alzheimer's sufferers is extremely small.

Everyone is exposed to aluminium because it is

very abundant in nature, but we do not know why it may cause damage in some people's brains. There is a theory that those at risk of Alzheimer's have some type of metabolic fault which causes them to accumulate aluminium but this has not been substantiated.

Most doctors specializing in Alzheimer's feel that there is no need to throw out aluminium saucepans or other utensils because the evidence for it leading to Alzheimer's is extremely slim. The latest advice is that Alzheimer's sufferers have nothing to gain from reducing aluminium intake. It seems that aluminium is only one of the environmental factors that may cause or accelerate the progress of the disease.

Q If aluminium can be ruled out, what else might cause Alzheimer's?

It is possible that there is no one, simple cause and never will be, any more than there is a single, simple cause of cancer. There may well be a genetic factor, in that the brains of some people are more susceptible to the kind of disorder and disintegration of Alzheimer's, but this has yet to be demonstrated. At the moment, there is a great deal of research into possible genetic factors, and this may or may not yield any information of importance in the future. Certainly, genetics is the most exciting research avenue into illness generally but, with Alzheimer's, there is no way of predicting who might succumb.

Viruses are another popular research field at the moment. Most viral infections, such as colds and influenza, develop and subside over a fairly short time. Some serious infections of the brain develop quickly but, in the more serious viral illnesses, the virus generally lies dormant in the system for years. The connection between genetics and viral infections is that people may be born with viruses in their systems which do not become apparent for many years. Some so-called 'slow' viruses are known to affect the brain and it has been postulated that Alzheimer's may fall into this category. The most likely cause of Alzheimer's is the agent responsible for Creutzfeldt-Jakob disease, which, in some cases, runs in families.

The most recent theory suggests that Alzheimer's results from an inherited malfunction of a protective brain protein. Dr Allen Roses of Duke University, USA, an Alzheimer's expert, formerly believed that the disease amounted to the brain simply wearing out in susceptible people. He has since discovered a protein, known as ApoE4, which seems to lack the ability to bind to another protein called tau. Alzheimer's patients have an excess of ApoE4.

Unbound tau, it seems, can damage neurons, and it seems as if people with ApoE4 are particularly prone to late-onset Alzheimer's. Dr Roses and his team are hoping that an ApoE4 substitute will eventually prevent the disease by binding to tau. But first, we need to know more about who might be at risk. There is not much point in medicating a whole nation against Alzheimer's when only a very few people may succumb to it. The cost alone would be prohibitive.

There may one day be an early test for Alzheimer's, but this is not likely to happen in the near future. And even if there were an early test, this would be of little use without some foolproof way of arresting the development of the disease.

Q Is there something wrong with the immune systems of Alzheimer's sufferers?

Many diseases associated with ageing occur because the immune system stops working efficiently. To function properly, the immune system must be able to recognize and destroy alien viruses, bacteria and cells; some diseases, for example cancer, occur because the body can no longer tell the difference between normal and abnormal tissue.

There is some evidence, albeit inconclusive, that Alzheimer's may be caused by an immune system dysfunction, which results in the build-up of β-amyloid, the protein responsible for destroying the brain cells of Alzheimer's sufferers.

If Alzheimer's is caused by a faulty immune system, even partly, this begs the question of what causes the immune system to become dysfunctional. It is certainly not related to the normal ageing processes, as not all elderly people get Alzheimer's.

Q Is there a connection with AIDS?

AIDS can affect the brain in a similar way to Alzheimer's disease. Early signs of AIDS are apathy, slowing down of mental processes and loss of memory and concentration, sometimes accompanied by mood disorder and paranoia. In the future an HIV antibody test may be required, to exclude AIDS, when Alzheimer's is being diagnosed.

Q Can Alzheimer's sufferers themselves understand the diagnosis?

The fact that Alzheimer's is being recognized increasingly earlier – although as we have seen, there is still no absolutely reliable diagnostic test – means that more people are having to face up to a positive diagnosis while they are still capable of understanding it. Ex-President Ronald Reagan recently announced that he probably has Alzheimer's, although the diagnosis must remain a matter of probability and opinion rather than fact until his brain is examined in a post-mortem examination.

Q Could a bang on the head cause Alzheimer's?

Some authorities have suggested that head injuries could spark off excess production of β-amyloid, the protein associated with brain deterioration in Alzheimer's sufferers. In 1991, British researchers examining the brains of road accident victims with head injuries found deposits of this protein similar to those which build up in the brains of Alzheimer's sufferers. Dr Gareth Roberts, the Alzheimer's expert who first proposed the head injury theory, believes that Alzheimer's may have a number of causes and that head injuries cannot be ruled out. A similar type of protein accumulation has been found in the brains of boxers who have become punch drunk.

Q **Could there be a dietary factor?**

There is an extremely controversial theory that meat eating could lead to Alzheimer's – a theory rejected by orthodox doctors and researchers.

Alzheimer's is known to have a connection with Creutzfeldt-Jakob Disease, the slow viral infection related to bovine spongiform encephalopathy (BSE or 'mad cow' disease).

Modern meat production methods, which involve feeding cows with protein from dead animals, including cows, can lead to BSE. It is suspected that cows, which are naturally herbivorous, begin to produce more β-amyloid protein when fed in this way. The protein accumulates in the brains of cows, causing the brains to become 'holey' like Aero chocolate bars.

Because BSE is diet-related, it is thought that Creutzfeldt-Jakob disease may be caused in a similar fashion, although there is no proof. Nevertheless it is worth considering whether brain degeneration diseases in human beings, in which there is a similar accumulation of β-amyloid protein, might also have dietary causes. It is possible that eating beef, veal, lamb and mutton containing abnormal proteins could trigger off a similar disease in human beings. At the moment, however, this is highly speculative.

It is not known whether vegetarians are at less risk of Alzheimer's than meat eaters but, certainly, the disease is not confined to meat eaters.

It has also been suggested that eating fruit stewed in aluminium pans may lead to Alzheimer's, because of its aluminium content, but evidence is inconclusive and flimsy.

2 Treatment Options

Q
What sort of questions will doctors ask when Alzheimer's is suspected?

With Alzheimer's, relatives, friends or partners almost always notice that there is something wrong long before the sufferer has any idea. Therefore, partners of sufferers are advised to talk to their doctor as soon as they suspect that memory loss and confusion have become permanent rather than temporary. It is possible that the problem is something other than Alzheimer's and it may be treatable.

The main symptom of Alzheimer's is always the same: loss of memory. Doctors will ask questions aimed at defining the exact extent of the memory loss and whether this has become noticeably worse over the previous few months.

Some people have always been forgetful so Alzheimer's should not be suspected just because the person is old. However, any dramatic changes in memory that are out of character, or out of previous character, may be significant. Your doctor may also ask whether the patient has suffered any kind of brain injury in the past, and whether drugs and alcohol are being taken excessively.

At this stage if your doctor suspects Alzheimer's, he or she will probably ask you to bring in the patient in order to carry out a complete physical examination. He or she may also order laboratory tests to screen for other illnesses, e.g. anaemia, cancer, infections or brain tumours. The doctor may carry out some psychological testing or refer the patient to a specialist in this. It may take some time before Alzheimer's is confirmed.

Q Will there one day be a drug to cure Alzheimer's?

The hope is that, one day, there will be a drug treatment effective for Alzheimer's but, so far, all attempts to find such a drug have been unsuccessful.

One of the problems with modern medicine is that the public is constantly being led to believe that an effective drug is just around the corner. In some cases, this has happened. For instance, until there were effective drugs to treat cystitis, sufferers used to die from the complaint. But, for many of today's highly complicated diseases, there seems to be no one simple drug which will cure the disease once and for all.

Research is going on all over the world to try and find an effective cure for cancer, AIDS, arthritis and heart disease but, so far, although certain medications can reduce symptoms and, in some cases, prolong life, they always seem to have either unacceptable side effects or prove completely ineffective after a promising start.

At the moment the quest for a drug for Alzheimer's seems to be following a similar pattern. Researchers and scientists have become excited about new drugs, only to find that either they help only a very small number of people, or the side effects become intolerable, and worse than the disease. The problem is to discover a way of generating new, healthy brain tissue and, at the moment, the best that science has so far come up with is some small amount of damage limitation.

Q How is research proceeding?

A team from Bristol University, UK, is synthesizing a nerve growth hormone, a naturally occurring protein thought to be the substance most likely to be able to halt or reverse the disease. Naturally, this substance occurs only in very small quantities, but it has now been produced by genetic engineering.

Once clinical trials have been completed, and the new substance receives ethical approval, the intention is to inject it into the brains of selected patients during neurosurgery. If the results prove successful, the Bristol team will try to develop a pill that can be more easily taken. Professor Gordon Wilcock, head of the Bristol team, believes that nerve growth hormone, or Nerve Growth Factor (NGF) as it is also known, constitutes a major breakthrough for Alzheimer's sufferers.

NGF was first identified in 1948 by Italian scientists, but its connection with Alzheimer's was not recognized until 1988. It was then discovered that NGF helped to keep alive some of the brain cells threatened with destruction by Alzheimer's. Professor Wilcock points out that, even when available in large quantities, the drug will only be effective in the early stages of the disease:

Nothing is going to take a very demented person and return them to normality. But eventually, in the cases of early diagnosis, we may be able to stop people getting worse and preserve them with a reasonable intellect.

What kind of drugs are available now?

There are a number of drugs which can treat the symptoms of Alzheimer's. The one which has caused most excitement in the medical world is tacrine (THA), currently the latest anti-cholinergic drug. This acts by blocking the enzyme involved in the breakdown of the acetylcholine in the brain. Acetylcholine is a neurotransmitter, i.e. it carries electrochemical signals from cell to cell, and it has been implicated in Alzheimer's.

Alzheimer's patients have been found to have low levels of acetylcholine in the brain and the hope has been that, by delaying the breakdown of acetylcholine, tacrine will also delay the mental deterioration.

The first medical paper on tacrine was published in The Lancet in 1991, when researchers at the Maudsley Hospital in London, UK, reported that the substance could delay deterioration by up to a year in Alzheimer's patients. After this study, further research seemed to show little if any benefit from tacrine. There is also concern that this drug could adversely affect the liver and, for this reason, it has been refused a licence in the UK. Tacrine was granted a licence in France in 1994 and has now been licensed in the USA, where there have been small improvements in some patients.

Other drugs under investigation have proved even less useful in the treatment of Alzheimer's and, although some have succeeded in reducing depression and improving mood, they have had no effect on the progress of the disease.

One of the major problems in developing drugs to treat Alzheimer's is that there is so little agreement on what causes the disease. All that is known so far are the effects and the fact that tangles and plaques characterize the condition.

As yet, no one knows what causes some people to produce too much β-amyloid protein. There may be a number of factors involved – a team at St Mary's Hospital, London, UK, showed that head injuries could trigger off amyloid deposits – and, so far, it is anyone's guess as to what they might be.

A very small number of people with Alzheimer's are genetically predisposed to producing too much of this protein and, so far, research suggests that all the brain abnormalities associated with Alzheimer's spring from excess β-amyloid. So perhaps an amyloid-reducing drug will prove to be the answer.

However, such a drug is not even on the drawing board as yet. Dr Gareth Roberts, of St Mary's Hospital Medical School, believes that, if the excess protein could be safely removed, progression of the disease could be halted. But how is the protein to be removed? And how can it be prevented from building up in the brains of sufferers?

A report in the Drug and Therapeutics Bulletin (May 1990) concluded that specific drugs for treating Alzheimer's were generally ineffective and that, although the disease process is now better understood than ever before, there have been no genuine therapeutic advances.

The final statement was that the best policy is to support carers as much as possible and to treat the mood and behaviour problems, as they arise, with other kinds of drugs.

Q **Are there any drugs that do any good?**

Although there are no drugs that will effect a cure, some drugs may be necessary to control the worst of the symptoms.

If the sufferer becomes very anxious, anxiety-reducing drugs may be prescribed. These will not affect the progress of the disease but may make day-to-day management easier. Tranquillizers may be prescribed for sufferers who become belligerent, aggressive or hostile. Night wandering, a common symptom of Alzheimer's, can be troublesome as well as dangerous and sedatives may be needed, if only so that others in the household can get some sleep. Cramps and seizures are also suffered by some Alzheimer's sufferers, usually in the later stages of the disease, and there are no effective drug treatments for these. Nor is there any surgery that will make any difference.

Drug treatment for reducing the symptoms of Alzheimer's is not a simple matter because, in the elderly, all strong drugs can have adverse side effects and drugs are not handled so well by the body systems. There may be Parkinsonian side effects and these, when added to Alzheimer's, can make the sufferer very difficult indeed.

Some drugs may cause muscular rigidity, stiffness and tremor. Tranquillizers, e.g. Valium, in very small doses, are probably the safest, but may make memory loss even worse. Tranquillizers can cause addiction but this is of little consequence in Alzheimer's sufferers.

Choosing and prescribing a drug regimen for an

Alzheimer's sufferer is not easy, because there are no drugs designed specifically for the disease; they are all meant for other purposes. Although one might imagine that there must be some drugs which can help, this does not seem to be the case with Alzheimer's. So far, nothing appears to work for long, or the side effects are too severe to make the drug regimen worth continuing.

Most doctors specializing in Alzheimer's suggest that any drugs which are taken should be administered only in very small doses, to see what happens. If there is some improvement, then the drugs may be continued. Most Alzheimer's patients are prescribed some kind of drug regimen at some stage, to alleviate symptoms and reduce the burden on the carers.

Q Are there any alternative or complementary treatments that work?

No claims made so far have yet stood up to investigation. There is an important basic difference between orthodox and alternative treatments. Conventional medical treatment is passive and depends on the doctor or surgeon giving pills or performing surgery; the patient puts nothing into the treatment.

In contrast, all alternative treatments demand input from the person being treated; i.e. the patient takes an active part in his or her care.

This presents us with the first difficulty in devising alternative treatments for Alzheimer's sufferers – patients can rarely look after themselves and usually, have no idea what is happening to them. Therefore they are unable to follow any kind of alternative regimen.

Nevertheless, because medical treatments and drugs have had such disappointing results, there have been a few attempts at alternative, i.e., non-conventional, treatments for Alzheimer's, but most experts believe they constitute quackery rather than any effective treatment.

The two principle alternative treatments are cortico-suppression and chelation therapy.

Cortico-suppression is based on the assumption that a special kind of hormone (adrenocortico-trophic hormone or ACTH) is produced to excess by Alzheimer's sufferers but there is no evidence of any kind to support this assumption and the treatment is ineffective.

Chelation therapy is widely recommended by

holistic and complementary clinics. This treatment is based on the theory that aluminium is contained in excess quantities in the brains of Alzheimer's patients, and that chelators – chemical compounds which remove certain metals from tissues – can remove this excess.

At the moment, scientific trials of chelation therapy are under way in the USA but, so far, no conclusions have been reached. Chelation therapy enjoyed a considerable vogue in the UK a few years ago but results did not stand up to the initial claims.

Chelation therapy for Alzheimer's sufferers could prove dangerous because chelators remove essential as well as non-essential minerals from the body. In particular, calcium and magnesium might be lost.

Another aspect of alternative treatments is their cost; financial difficulties are common among families facing Alzheimer's.

Although some treatments, such as massage, aromatherapy and relaxation techniques, may help patients to feel better, there is no way that any of them can halt the march of the disease. The best advice is to avoid any alternative or complementary treatments where there is no rationale for their use in this particular disease.

3 Caring for Alzheimer's Sufferers

Q Can Alzheimer's patients look after themselves?

In the early stages, yes. Before long, however, according to the progress of the disease, all sufferers will need round-the-clock care and skilled nursing. Unfortunately there is no alternative and families and carers should prepare themselves for this eventuality. It is no good hoping that this will not be necessary, or that the disease will arrest itself at an early stage. One of the saddest aspects of the condition is that it only gets worse.

Q How are sufferers best looked after?

Over the past few years, great strides have been made in the humane understanding of Alzheimer's sufferers and their management – the word used when there is no effective treatment available. Above all, carers should learn in advance all about the progression of the disease so that they can be prepared, and so that the shocks are minimized.

It is very distressing to see a much-loved relative gradually sink into Alzheimer's and carers may be tempted to imagine that there will be improvement if enough loving care is given. Unfortunately, this is not the case and, in many ways, it is a thankless task to look after somebody suffering from this disease.

Carers should always be aware of just how much of the sufferer's mental capacity remains, and how that capacity compares with what he or she was like, say, a year ago. In the early stages of the disease, sufferers may realize that they have some degree of memory loss, but the tendency is to minimize or deny it. When this happens, carers should not confront the sufferer with the truth, as it will do no good, but they should try to anticipate when the worst aspects of memory loss and forgetfulness are likely to occur.

It is tempting to imagine that all Alzheimer's sufferers eventually become the same but this is not the case. Reactions to the disease, and the disease itself, vary considerably and the only thing to do is to remind yourself of the patient's personality. For a long time, some aspects of the previous personality will remain.

Although Alzheimer's sufferers commonly deny

that there is anything wrong, so do relatives and carers. Because there is still a stigma attached to an illness affecting mental capacity, relatives and carers may also deny and minimize the disease – and try to continue as if there is nothing wrong. Doctors find that partners are often the last to admit that a dementing disease has set in; they try to persuade themselves that it isn't happening, or to find other explanations of the signs.

It is often grown-up children, neighbours or other relatives who are the first to spot, or at least to say, that something is wrong. Partners often try to put the signs down to inevitable ageing. The best and bravest thing to do is to admit the problem and then become as expert as possible in dealing with it. Facing up to it is often half the battle.

Q If I suspect that somebody close to me may have Alzheimer's, what should I do?

The first thing to do is to seek medical advice. Although there are no effective medical treatments, this does not mean that there is nothing the medical profession can do to help. You should not try to cope entirely on your own and should bear in mind that often a problem shared is a problem halved.

Tell your doctor about the signs that you have spotted and ask for an opinion. If you are a partner, possibly the most difficult thing to accept is that there will be a gradual deterioration and that you will eventually lose, in any meaningful sense, the person who means the most to you.

If Alzheimer's is confirmed, the first thing to do is to try and persuade the affected person to give up the tasks that are now beyond him or her, for instance driving a car. This is not easy, as most people imagine they are perfectly fit behind the wheel long after they are not actually safe on the road. Doctors can help by persuading the affected person that it may be better not to drive in future. Some doctors suggest hiding the keys if the sufferer persists in wanting to drive.

It may also be necessary for the sufferer to retire early from work, especially if the work involves dealing with dangerous or delicate items. In many cases, the main carer may also have to consider giving up work, because before long it will be impossible to leave the sufferer alone.

A lot of expertise about Alzheimer's and all kinds of local clubs and societies, holidays and help are available which can alleviate the burden on the primary carer. There are day centres, places where there are experts in looking after Alzheimer's sufferers, and all options should be explored.

For example there is a day centre, in Abingdon, UK, which receives a local-authority grant, where sufferers can go for 4 days a week. The centre is staffed by paid and voluntary workers, all skilled at coping with Alzheimer's patients. Although many sufferers have little idea what is happening, they pass the time by playing snakes and ladders, although they usually forget which side they are on, and by holding sing-songs. Rosemary Varney, who works at the centre, says that most people don't sing in tune, and few remember the words, but this doesn't matter. The important thing is that patients who have forgotten how to talk can still remember how to sing. More day centres like this one are being set up all the time, and they can be a godsend to primary carers. There are about 80 support groups for Alzheimer's sufferers in the UK, and these are worth investigating at an early stage.

Q Should I help the sufferer to keep the brain active?

Most experts believe that this is pointless and counterproductive. It can be tempting, in the early stages, to try to stimulate the sufferer in order to keep the brain working. But remember that the brain is gradually deteriorating and that sufferers forget because their brain can no longer function to its full capacity.

As more of the brain's function becomes lost, sufferers will gradually withdraw from stimulating activities and give up all hobbies. There is no point in trying to interest them again; they have withdrawn because their brains can no longer cope with the task.

As Alzheimer's progresses, there will also be a gradual withdrawal from all social activities. Social occasions become increasingly difficult for sufferers to cope with, so carers should keep the number of new faces and new occasions to a minimum.

Take note when sufferers become anxious. Anxiety is a major symptom of Alzheimer's and a sign that the brain is being overloaded. Sufferers may become increasingly anxious about ordinary or everyday tasks, such as washing up, getting dressed, shaving. When this happens, the best plan is to persuade them to give up control of this activity to someone else. In some cases, it makes sense to let the sufferer carry on for as long as possible, provided that others are not adversely affected. Nevertheless, carers should always be on the lookout for things which cause undue anxiety.

Most sufferers come to value what is safe and familiar, so carers should limit the amount of new material which can be taken on board. It is best to maintain a routine whereby everything, as far as possible, follows a set pattern. Most doctors advise making everything predictable. All disruptions to this routine should be kept to a minimum.

Doctors also advise keeping the home environment as familiar as possible, for as long as the sufferer continues to live at home. Don't rearrange furniture and don't let newspapers, magazines or litter accumulate, as this will worry the sufferer.

Sometimes when Alzheimer's strikes, people consider moving to a new home: perhaps a bungalow or sheltered housing. This is almost always a mistake. The less new information to be assimilated, the better. New surroundings can make Alzheimer's sufferers unduly anxious because they cannot retain existing information, let alone new information, and there will be increasing anxiety coupled with a decreased ability to reason and be logical. If a move is essential, it is best made as early on in the disease as possible, while there is still some memory and reasoning power left, and while the sufferer can appreciate and understand what is going on.

Q What about going to the toilet? Can this be a problem?

Yes, certainly. Some sufferers become incontinent or may suffer from constipation. If this becomes a problem it may be necessary to administer a suitable laxative or other drug.

Eventually, there will be loss of bladder and bowel control. Coping at home can then become difficult and it is often this factor which leads carers to the decision that the sufferer needs to go into a nursing home. There are no easy answers but it may help to be prepared for the inevitable and to seek the prior advice of your doctor.

Q Do sufferers retain an interest in sex?

As the disease progresses, all interest in sex, as in other activities, will gradually be lost. Although some sufferers may start to use uncharacteristically sexual language and appear overly concerned with sexual matters, understand that this is because of the disease, not for any other reason.

However, it can be extremely distressing when

sufferers accuse their partners of having affairs or of being adulterous behind their backs without foundation, although, after such accusations, the sufferers usually become remorseful and weepy. Generally the only way to cope with such incidents is to ignore them. They will pass, mean nothing, and have nothing to do with any real fears on the part of the sufferer. In a few cases, however, persisting delusions of infidelity may lead to violence.

Q Are there any other physical signs of decline?

Because the brain is deteriorating rapidly, sight and hearing may become noticeably impaired. Normally, although these faculties gradually diminish with age, memory can make good the loss. With Alzheimer's, as memory is lost, they may appear to deteriorate rapidly although there is no physical degeneration of the eyes and ears.

Because of the impairment of these senses, sufferers may become very anxious about light and sound. It may be necessary to have lights turned up full all the time, even at night, to allay this anxiety. Some experts advise installing fluorescent lamps as this is the most intense form of lighting available and can be run relatively cheaply.

It may help to keep a radio or tape playing very familiar songs and music. Remember that Alzheimer's sufferers like what they are used to; unfamiliar songs and music will make them unduly anxious.

Hearing aids are not much help to Alzheimer's sufferers and again, are something new to get used and will cause anxiety. Researchers into the disease believe that it is just about impossible for sufferers to become accustomed to a hearing aid. Any new, distracting noises should be avoided whenever possible.

To sum up, the best way of caring for an Alzheimer's sufferer at home is to keep things as calm, familiar and safe as possible, and to avoid any unusual distractions of any kind.

Q **Many old people are nervous about unfamiliar and new things. How do Alzheimer's patients differ?**

Alzheimer's patients can cope for a long time with the familiar; it is the new which worries them, and this applies to new people as much as new surroundings or new furniture. This also applies to many old people but, with Alzheimer's sufferers, it is much more than just a preference;

they become frightened and nervous at the prospect of anything new. This can put an enormous burden on carers but whatever can be done to minimize anxiety-causing events will make everyone involved more comfortable and serene.

Because Alzheimer's sufferers lose their curiosity and do not move around much, they are at no great risk from ordinary household hazards. Nevertheless, a few sensible precautions may be in order, for example installing a smoke alarm in case they forget to turn off ovens or fires, and having locks installed which can be opened from both sides of the door, so that they do not get locked in the bathroom.

Wandering may become a problem, so it is a good idea to sew name and address labels into clothing. Eventually, as the disease progresses, the sufferer will need round-the-clock care and will have to be dressed, taken to the toilet, washed and fed.

Unfortunately, there is little that can be done to prevent this, and it is as well to be prepared. If the sufferer lives long enough, it is unavoidable. Doctors treating Alzheimer's sufferers have noted that the primary carer, usually the partner, frequently tries to carry on alone for far too long and is often too proud to ask for help from neighbours, friends or family.

Eventually, however, constant care will be necessary; no one can cope alone and professional help will be required.

The best thing that sufferers and carers can do at an early stage is to join the Alzheimer's Disease Society. There are many local branches and many countries now have Alzheimer's Associations. These can give excellent practical help and advice on many matters, including care and nursing homes, drugs and research.

Q What should I tell children, relatives and friends about the problem?

If there are children living in the same house as an Alzheimer's sufferer, they will certainly be aware that something is going on before they are told. It is always best to be truthful and to give as much accurate information as they are able to understand. Some doctors working with Alzheimer's patients feel that children are often better at accepting the condition than adults, who have higher expectations of fellow adults.

One problem is embarrassment in the presence of their friends and, in this case, if children prefer not to brings friends home because they might laugh at the elderly relative, it is best not to insist. If the Alzheimer's sufferer has to go into a nursing home, children may not want to visit. They should not be forced into visiting, and young children in particular should certainly not visit when the patient has long ceased to recognize them or remember who they are. When this happens, there is simply no point and the encounter is unpleasant for all concerned.

So far as family members and neighbours are concerned, it is also best to be truthful and admit that your relative is suffering from Alzheimer's. The more open people can be about the condition, the less shame will be attached to it.

It is not always easy for other relatives, neighbours and friends to appreciate just how difficult it can be to look after an Alzheimer's sufferer, and you may be accused of not having done enough, or of upsetting the patient. Here, you must bear in mind that others may feel guilty, they may not understand the condition fully and, in any case, you are not responsible for their reactions.

But whatever their reaction might be, it is always best not to try to hide the Alzheimer's or other dementing condition, or to pretend that everything is the same as before. If other relatives feel that not enough is being done, ask them to look after the sufferer for a few days, just to see what is involved. Onlookers rarely have any accurate idea of how difficult it can be to look after an Alzheimer's sufferer when the condition is rapidly worsening.

Q Will an Alzheimer's sufferer always need hospital care?

Eventually, yes. There comes a time when, with the best will in the world, sufferers can no longer be looked after at home. This presents many problems, chief of which is finding a hospital or home that will take an Alzheimer's patient and is set up for this kind of expert care.

Q Do ordinary hospitals take Alzheimer's patients?

Not usually. In the UK, National Health Service (NHS) hospitals only take people suffering from Alzheimer's if they also have some other physical illness requiring hospital treatment. Most are just not equipped for this kind of long-term care.

Although the NHS has a responsibility to care for Alzheimer's patients, in many cases in the UK, this responsibility has been transferred to local authorities and the kind of care available under their auspices varies greatly from area to area. Nor do private hospitals usually offer the kind of care that Alzheimer's patients need. Moreover, the cost is prohibitive and cannot be met through private insurance schemes.

In the United States, few people with dementias are in state hospitals and those who are are mostly patients considered too disruptive to be cared for in a nursing home. Medicaid funds nursing home care for Alzheimer's patients who qualify for Supplemental Security Income. State hospitals can be paid through Medicare, as long as the hospital is accredited and provides proper care for dementia patients.

Other care options in the United States are Veterans' Administration Hospitals, although these cater mainly for ex-service people, and private hospitals which do not usually offer extended nursing care for demential patients because of the extremely high cost.

The other factor that must be taken into consideration is that Alzheimer's sufferers only thrive

– in so far as they thrive at all – on what is familiar. Sudden hospitalization can bring about an acute deterioration in their condition although, if there is a physical condition, such as a heart attack or broken hip, sufferers will need hospital treatment. It can be heartbreaking to see how quickly their condition deteriorates when extra stresses, such as seeing strange people, being in a strange and frightening environment, are added and behaviour can become out of character. It is not unusual for Alzheimer's sufferers to become confused and distressed, to start wandering or even to become verbally abusive with hospital staff and relatives who come to visit. It must be borne in mind that this is an aspect of the disease, not deliberate behaviour.

Q What financial provisions should be made?

Because eventually, caring for somebody with Alzheimer's becomes a 7-day-a-week, 24-hour-a-day job, with no time for anything else much in between, including earning a living, the Alzheimer's Society recommend going into all the options at a very early stage, before drastic decisions have to be taken. Whatever the course of the disease, carers must assume that, at some stage, the sufferer will become completely incapable of handling financial matters; this always happens.

One of the problems, of course, is knowing how much financial, or other, competence remains with the sufferer. In the early stages, there may be hostility and aggression, suspicion and mistrust if he or she is advised to hand over responsibility for financial affairs.

One of the things the Society strongly advises is to arrange for an Enduring Power of Attorney (EPA). Ideally, everyone should, in this way, appoint someone to manage their financial or other affairs, if the need arises. This legal device gives the partner, or other carer, authorization to carry out all financial matters and it must be done while the sufferer is still completely of sound mind or it is not valid. If there is no close family member, this task may fall to a neighbour, but it must be done because, once Alzheimer's strikes, there must be someone available who can take decisions on behalf of the sufferer.

The EPA should be taken out as soon as there are any signs of memory loss. The Society can provide all all the details and advice required.

The sufferer must be able to understand all the

implications, and it is best to draw up the document with a solicitor. It is better, say the Society, than waiting for the next stage, which involves going to court and becomes much more expensive and complicated.

The other important matter which needs attention is that of a will. Carers should find out whether a will has been made, and, if not, try to persuade the sufferer to make one before irreversible confusion sets in. If there is a will, carers should make sure the sufferer understands all the implications and does not want any changes made.

It may also be necessary at a fairly early stage to obtain a power of attorney tax form, so that a responsible person can sign and deal with the sufferer's income tax.

Although all this may seem like interfering, and nobody wants to be accused of busybodying, there is no sense in hoping the Alzheimer's will go away. A great deal of confusion and many problems arise when families refuse to face these matters. Sometimes, the family has no choice but to exercise financial control and to obtain this control by legal means; bills and mortgages still have to be paid, and savings and financial transactions managed.

Financial matters do not go away just because somebody is suffering from Alzheimer's, and they often present the most enduring and difficult problems to deal with. There may also be bitter disputes between family members about who is best equipped to deal with the financial affairs and who is most trustworthy. Other family members may accuse carers of trying to get their hands on a mother's money, or persuading her to alter her will when not of sound mind.

In many ways, Alzheimer's can split families apart and it seems to be the most sensible solution for the person providing the bulk of the care to be the one to handle money and other such matters. If this person is not competent, or is dishonest, then in a way, that is too bad; few people want to take over responsibility for an Alzheimer's sufferer.

Usually, the main task of caring for Alzheimer's sufferers goes to the partners and it is vital that they understand what is involved as they, too, may not be in the best of health. If in doubt, they should get expert advice as soon as possible, or ask a competent family member to help. They should not try to cope alone when they do not know what to do for the best. There are experts around: use them.

Can the Social Services help ?

Theoretically, yes. In the UK, the type and quality of care available varies according to area. The best thing to do, as soon as memory loss becomes apparent but before the disease gets to an advanced stage, is to enquire as to what services are available and what their cost might be. In some areas services are free, while in other areas you will have to pay for nursing, meals-on-wheels, home helps, etc.

In the United States, the social service departments at county court offices can provide information on services available.

It must be borne in mind that, eventually, an Alzheimer's sufferer will be beyond the care of relatives and friends, however willing they may be to help. Expertise is needed as the disease progresses.

There are day centres which relieve some of the burden on the primary carer but these vary greatly from area to area. Some provide day care which enables the carer to go out to work, while others provide facilities for only a few hours a week.

It is always extremely difficult to find carers who

will come into the home and who are able to offer good nursing skills. The fact of the matter is that few people want to care for advanced Alzheimer's sufferers; it is a thankless task. In practice, carers often fail to turn up, they want days off, holidays and sick days, and few are willing to stay overnight or care for an incontinent patient.

This may sound distressing and unhelpful, but it is the stark reality of the situation facing those who want to continue to care for their Alzheimer's relatives at home.

Q What about nursing homes?

This is a difficult area and there are no easy solutions. If the standard of day care in your area is excellent, you may be able to cope without the sufferer going into a nursing home, but this cannot be guaranteed. Not all nursing homes are equipped to care for Alzheimer's sufferers and those that are may be extremely expensive.

Here is novelist Margaret Forster's experience of caring for a relative who developed Alzheimer's:

In the five years our family cared for my mother-in-law, we spent £42,000. The money was spent on relieving myself, my husband and most of all my sister-in-law, on whom the brunt fell. We had a team of five helpers, all paid by the hour, so that we could all work some part of the day.

This 'team' broke up all the time. By the stage that my mother-in-law was not only incontinent but falling out of bed every night, all night, we were unable to find anyone willing to cover the nights we could not. So we were defeated.

We thought, in our innocence, that we could find a lovely home for which, if necessary, we would pay through the nose. We failed to find one. By the time we started looking, my mother-in-law was too far along the road to complete helplessness for any 'good' home to take her.

So she went into the psycho-geriatric ward of a State mental hospital.

In her article in the *Observer* newspaper, from which this extract was taken, Margaret Forster points out that, although the care her mother-in-law received in the State mental hospital was not good, what was the alternative? Home helps, meals-on-wheels, grants for rubber sheets – none of these, she found, went anywhere near helping anyone care for an advanced Alzheimer's sufferer in their own home.

For Margaret Forster – and don't forget that she and her husband, the writer Hunter Davies, are successful, rich, sophisticated and articulate people who could, surely, make a system work for them if anyone could – there was simply nothing to be done.

Her conclusions are stark. Either those in the last stages of Alzheimer's should be helped to die or they must be kept alive in conditions which give them at least some semblance of dignity. She now feels that both sufferers and carers are treated with callous disregard – possibly because of the stigma still attached to illnesses which affect the brain and mental functioning.

Margaret Forster believes that wards like those which took in her mother-in-law should not exist, and she made a plea in her article for hospice-style establishments where sufferers might be cared for humanely in a warm, loving atmosphere. In her case, not even the availability of large sums of money could make any difference – there were just no nursing homes which would take a case as advanced as that of her mother-in-law.

Nevertheless, there are nursing homes available which specialize in the care of Alzheimer's patients. In these places, skilled nursing care is provided by registered and qualified nurses who know how to look after dementia patients. Occupational therapy may be provided and there are attempts to interest the patients in daily life and routine.

Perhaps the lesson to be learned from Margaret Forster's experience is this: don't continue to cope at home until the patient needs round-the-clock care. Make enquiries about nursing homes before this stage has been reached, so that a good home will take the patient before the very worst of the disease has manifested itself.

Q But aren't these nursing homes very expensive?

Yes, they are. Those who are very poor, who have no savings and do not own their home may be fortunate enough for the local authority to pay for such a nursing home. Most people, however, will not fall into this category and one hears terrible stories of people's houses being taken away, savings being eroded and stark poverty being faced to pay for nursing-home care. Also, very often, the primary carer will have to give up his or her job to care for the patient, thus making the financial situation even worse.

A story in the *Daily Mail* in June 1993 illustrated what can happen to people whose partners develop Alzheimer's.

Mrs Emma Sturdy-Morton and her husband, who had been a career diplomat, moved to a house in Sussex on his retirement. They had planned to live on his pension and what they had managed to save over the years. Then he was diagnosed as having Alzheimer's and his condition deteriorated rapidly. He soon became beyond home care, and doctors recommended that his wife put him in a suitable nursing home. In 1993, this was going to cost at least £400 a week.

It is the case in the UK that any savings over £8000 (in 1995) can be taken to pay for nursing-home care.

Mrs Sturdy-Morton was informed by her local council that all her assets, including her husband's occupational pension, would be taken to pay for his medical care. She would have no income whatever. When she asked what she was expected to live on, she was told to apply for income support.

Others contact the Alzheimer's Disease Society regularly with stories like this one, and the Society has confirmed that they are not exaggerated.

The financial situation in the UK in respect of caring for someone with Alzheimer's is as follows. Until 1 April 1993, a number of National Health Service (NHS) beds were available to take patients with Alzheimer's but, under the new NHS Trust guidelines, the number of continuing care beds has been cut and patients are being increasingly transferred to the private sector. Also, Social Security payments made to individuals towards the cost of residential homes are now means-tested.

The net effect is that, the longer an Alzheimer's patient lives, the poorer the carer or partner will become. Carers and partners are now being forced into penury and, eventually, may have to claim State benefits. The state is therefore paying any-way, just to keep these people alive.

Social Services departments will make a contri-bution towards the fees of sufferers who are considered to be beyond home care and in need of nursing-home care.

These contributions are calculated by a means test, in which all income and capital, including the home, and again, any savings over about £8000 are taken into account.

Social services can claim 100 per cent of a husband's pension, leaving the wife with nothing to live on. If it is the wife who suffers from Alzheimer's the situation may be slightly better financially as, normally, only 50 per cent of the man's pension would be allocated to his wife.

The non-working wives of men who contract Alzheimer's are the most badly affected although, as we have seen, Alzheimer's is no more common in men than women. But a wife who has no income of her own and relies on her husband's pension (as Alzheimer's is basically a disease of old age, most people affected will be retired or near retirement) will risk losing all the money she has if her husband has to go into a nursing home. There have been several cases of women whose husband's pension has all been earmarked to pay for his nursing home care.

One case that came to light was of a woman

whose sister had to go into residential care after a diagnosis of Alzheimer's. This woman, who had given up her job to look after her sister, discovered that the Social Services had claimed half the house, which she owned jointly with her sister. The woman was forced to sell the house and did not have enough money left to buy another one.

Eventually, there will be very few people who can afford long-term care in a nursing home. Margaret Forster (see page 85) expressed gratitude that her mother-in-law lived for only 5 years after being admitted to a State geriatric mental home. She could have lived on for another 10 years and, if she had been in a private home, this would have made a huge hole in even the largest income. Even so, the family had to find over £40,000 to pay helpers to care for her mother-in-law – hardly a tiny sum.

Another woman, whose widowed mother has Alzheimer's, is having to pay over £500 a week for a nursing home and, in order to raise this money, she has had to sell her mother's house. As her mother is in her early 70s, she could live for another 10 years. At present prices, this would mean an outlay of £250,000 – and her mother will never get better. Not only that, but she sees her inheritance vanishing daily, all spent on care for a woman whose condition will never improve, who no longer knows her, but who could live on for many more years.

There are no easy answers to the problems arising from Alzheimer's but, for many people, the spending of huge sums of money, loss of income and job, and possibly house, are among the hardest aspects to take. It is not surprising that people feel bitter about the way their hard-won savings become eroded by having to pay for the care of people with a disease of this type.

In a country with no welfare state, there would be no choice but many people feel that, as everyone compulsorily pays, one way or another, for a health service, then dementia patients should be properly looked after by the state. The Alzheimer's Disease Society believes that it is unrealistic to expect the welfare services to pay for everything, and for carers and families to make no contribution at all, but, under the present system, everyone pays considerable sums into a health service which then lets them down when they need it most.

No one wants to deny a loved one all the care available but, as Margaret Forster pointed out, there are just not the people, the money or the facilities to look after Alzheimer's sufferers the way they need to be looked after without enormous financial and personal drains on the carers.

Q Suppose a nursing home is the only option left, how do I find a good one?

Nursing homes need careful evaluation. You must remember that these homes are usually run for profit, and often, a group of nursing homes will be owned by a company. This does not mean that they do not provide a good service but, when it comes to caring for old people suffering from dementia, good staff are very hard to find. On the whole, it is not a job that people are clamouring to do.

The best thing is to join the Alzheimer's Disease Society, if you have not already done so, and to order their literature about what to look for in a nursing home and what exists in your particular area. Then look at several before making any decision.

When assessing the suitability of a home ask yourself the following questions. Is the home pleasant and clean? Are all areas well lit? Do residents have their own bedrooms or, if they are shared, how many are there to a room? What are the meals like? What is the general atmosphere in the dining room? Do the staff seem cheerful and positive? Are the nurses doing their best to interact with the residents? What kind of activities are encouraged? Take a good look at the residents. Do they look clean and well cared for? Are some of them smiling? Do they seem happy, given their condition?

It is especially important to know that residents are being well cared for when nursing homes cost up to £500 a week, or more if specially skilled nursing care is needed. (Some relatives have been appalled at the quality of care when they go to visit, finding that hair hasn't been washed, clean clothes haven't been put on, and the bedrooms have not been cleaned. Although this may be more distressing to visitors than residents, it is all part of humane care.)

It is also essential to do some research, bearing in mind that Alzheimer's patients need special, round-the-clock care. What is the ratio of staff to patients? Are the nurses all qualified, or does the home employ casual help? Ask also about specific medical care and what happens about prescription medicines, visiting and occupational therapy.

Q Do health insurance policies cover Alzheimer's?

The best advice here is to ask the sufferer, at an early stage of the disease, what health care insurance he or she may have and to take a careful look at the policy. It is unlikely that provision will be made for long-term care of people with Alzheimer's. If the sufferer is employed, he or she may be covered for illness or disability for a year by a company insurance plan. However, no policy will cover looking after a disabled person for years on end. Most health insurance policies state in the small print that illnesses such as progressive dementia, which have no time limit, are not covered. Therefore, once a person has developed Alzheimer's, he or she will probably no longer be insurable.

All other insurance policies, e.g. life insurance, should also be checked to see what the conditions are. If a diagnosis of Alzheimer's is made at an early stage, it may be possible for the family to keep life insurance policies in force.

Here again, the best people to contact are the Alzheimer's Disease Society, which has extensive experience in dealing with these matters. As every case is different, it is impossible to give general advice, other than to deal with all these matters at the earliest stage practicable.

It is a good idea to ask the sufferer about insurance policies of all kinds once there are definite signs of memory loss. Even if Alzheimer's is not diagnosed, it is still wise to check all policies carefully, contacting the insurance companies if anything seems unclear.

Above all, don't be panicked into buying new policies when illness strikes; the premiums will be expensive and cover may not be all that good.

Also check what pension and retirement and any disability allowances may be payable, especially if the patient has to retire early from work because of progressive illness. Also check with Social Security what disability, care allowance or other benefits may be forthcoming.

Q What is the future for sufferers from Alzheimer's and other progressive dementias?

There is no doubt that great strides have been made over the past few decades in understanding illnesses which affect the brain. During the 1950s, hardly anything was known about the structure of the brain, even though Alzheimer's was identified nearly 100 years ago. We now know far more about how the brain works, which chemical messengers are involved, and why and how things may go wrong. However, although much progress has been made, there is still no effective treatment for Alzheimer's sufferers. The most encouraging advances have been in the ways in which we regard the illness and sufferers can be looked after, rather than in any high-technology breakthroughs.

So far, studies and trials on drug treatments have proved disappointing, with no effective treatment even on the horizon. All the drugs which have been developed to deal with Alzheimer's and other dementias have too many side effects, are too difficult to administer, or benefit only a very small number of people – or all three. The hope is that, if the disease can be diagnosed at an early enough stage, there may be a drug which halts or slows down the decline.

Nor have scientists come very far with understanding the causes of Alzheimer's. At one time it seemed as though aluminium might be the major culprit, but that theory is becoming less likely in the light of new studies. If there is a genetic component, there is little we can do about our genetic inheritance. At the moment, the only 'treatment' which can be offered for genetically inherited diseases is to diagnose them in utero and then offer an abortion. This is happening with Down's syndrome and with muscular dystrophy. With cancers which have a genetic element, e.g. some breast cancers, the only treatment is mastectomy. It seems as if some new breakthrough is needed in the treatment of Alzheimer's, as all the avenues so far explored have been disappointing.

For the time being, we need to concentrate on the care of Alzheimer's patients and, particularly, to lighten the burden on primary carers. As yet, Alzheimer's is a terrible blow for all concerned: for the sufferer, for whom there is no cure or preventive treatment, and for the family who have to cope, often at terrible financial and emotional cost to themselves.

As Margaret Forster said in her Observer article, we need more hospice-type establishments where sufferers from advanced dementias can be looked after with some dignity and without carers suffering the dreadful financial losses which are so often the case at the moment.

In the past, sufferers would not have lived very long after contracting Alzheimer's disease. Now, with proper nutrition and greater understanding of the disease, they can live for many years, getting gradually worse, more forgetful and eventually losing touch with the world altogether.

If, with present knowledge and research, there is still little that can be done for Alzheimer's sufferers, let us at least try to lift the burden on those heroic family members who try to care for them. After all, it is the family who bear the brunt of the suffering, rather than the patient, who is unaware of what is going on.

Doctors in the UK have developed a genetic test which can now predict the severity of Alzheimer's in people with Down's syndrome who have already shown symptoms of the disease. The test is adapted from technology used for DNA fingerprinting and, as yet, is available only to Down's syndrome sufferers. The hope is that, in the future, the test, performed via amniocentesis, will be universally available so that the likelihood of Alzheimer's in later life can be predicted before birth.

The research was conducted by Dr Gareth Roberts, an Alzheimer specialist, and a team at Charing Cross Hospital, London. The test does not constitute a cure, nor is it preventative, but it may in future give a clearer idea of how fast the disease will progress, how bad it will become and what care and treatment may be required. Of course, tests of this kind open up all kinds of ethical issues, such as who gives consent for the test, and what do you do with the knowledge once you have it?

Dr Claire Royston, one of the scientists who developed this test, said: 'At present there is no cure for Alzheimer's. Our research could mean that doctors, carers and others will be able to improve the quality of life of both the person with the disease and their carer. As treatment becomes available over the next few years doctors could use this test to choose which treatment might be the best option for an individual.'

The race is on to find a cure – but still no one really knows how the β-amyloid plaques form in the first place. Once this has been established there must just be a chance that a drug to prevent this formation might be developed. But whether it will be safe, with no undue side effects, and whether it really will halt the progress of Alzheimer's, remains to be seen.

Scientists all over the world are now working dedicatedly on research projects to improve the lot of those who develop Alzheimer's disease. Let us also hope that, before long, a way is found of alleviating the burden on all those who have to cope with this devastating and irreversible disease.

Useful Addresses

United Kingdom

Alzheimer's Disease Society
Gordon House
10 Greencote Place
London SW1P 1PH
Tel. 0171 306 0606

Alzheimer's Disease Society of
Ireland
St John of God
Stillorgan
Co. Dublin
N. Ireland
Tel. 3531 288 1282

Alzheimer's Disease Society of
Scotland,
33 Castle Street
Edinburgh
Scotland
Tel. 0131 220 6155

The Mental Health Foundation
37 Mortimer Street
London W1N 8JU
Tel. 0171 580 0145

Australia

Alzheimer's Disease and Related
Disorders (ADARDS)
PO Box 51
North Ryde
NSW 2113
Tel. 611 878 4466

Canada

Alzheimer's Society of Canada
1320 Yonge Street, Suite 302
Toronto
Ontario MJ4T 1X2
Tel. 416 925 3552

New Zealand

Alzheimer's Disease and Related
Disorders (ADARDS)
Box 2828
Christchurch
Tel. 03 651 590

USA

Alzheimer's Disease International
70 East Lake Street
Chicago
Illinois 60601-5997
Tel. 312 853 3060

South Africa

Alzheimer's Disease and Related
Disorders (ADARDS)
PO Box 81183
Parkhurst
Johannesburg 2120
Tel. 011 782 7586

References

Burningham, S. (1989) Not On Your Own. Penguin.

Disability Alliance (1995) Disability Rights Handbook 1994/5.

Horwood, J. (1994) Caring: How to Cope. Health Education Authority.

Mace, N. & Rabins, P. (1992) The 36-Hour Day. Headway Hodder and Stoughton.

Murphy, E. (1993) Dementia and Illness in Older People. A Practical Guide. Papermac.

Wilcock, A. (1990) Living with Alzheimer's Disease. Penguin.

Woods, R. T. (1991) Alzheimer's Disease, Coping with a Living Death. Souvenir Press.

Index

Index

financial problems 80–3, 88–94
fluorescent lights 73
forgetfulness 26, 31, 54, 66
Forster, Margaret 85–8, 92, 93–4, 99
friends, telling about Alzheimer's 77–8

genetic engineering, nerve growth hormone 56
genetic factors 30, 45, 47–8, 59, 98–9
genetic tests 41, 100–1
growth hormone 56–7

Hayworth, Rita 12, 13–14
head injuries 51–2, 59
health insurance 79, 96–7
hearing aids 74
hearing problems 73–4
heart disease 36, 56
high blood pressure 36
HIV 50
home environment 71
    safety 75
home helps 86–7
hormones:
    cortico-suppression 63
    nerve growth 56–7
hospices 99
hospital care 78–80
hostility 27
Huntington's disease 38
hydrocephalus 38
hyperactivity 28
hypodermic syringes 46

immune system 8, 49–50
income support 90
income tax 82

incontinence 72
infidelity, delusions of 73
influenza 37, 48
inheritance of Alzheimer's *see* genetic factors
injuries, head 51–2, 59
insurance, medical 79, 96–7
IQ (intelligence quotient tests) 39–40

kidney dialysis 46

labels, name and address 75
The Lancet 58
laxatives 72
Lewy body disease 39
life insurance 96
lights 73
local authorities 79, 88, 89–90
locks 75
long-term memory 23–4, 31

'mad cow' disease 52
magnesium, chelation therapy 64
massage 64
Maudsley Hospital, London 58
meals-on-wheels 87
means tests 91
meat eating 52–3
Medicaid 79
medical insurance 79, 96–7
Medicare 79
memory loss:
    in Alzheimer's 23–4, 25–7, 31, 42, 54, 66
    forgetfulness 26, 31, 54, 66
    long-term memory 23–4, 31
    other causes 25–6
    short-term memory 23–4
    tests 40

Index